LESLIE NADON

D1615906

THE

HINDU-YOGI

BREATHING EXERCISES

A System of Physical, Mental and Soul Development

BY THE ORIENTAL OCCULT SCIENCE OF RHYTHMIC AND VIBRATIONAL BREATHING

By YOGI RAMACHARAKA

Author of "Science of Breath;" "Fourteen Lessons in Yogi Philosophy and Oriental Occultism;" "Advanced Course, Etc.;" "Hatha Yoga, or, The Yogi Philosophy of Physical Well-Being;" "A Series of Lessons in Raja Yoga;" Etc., Etc.

ISBN 0-911662-62-6

CONTENTS

CHAPTER I.
WHO ARE THE YOGIS?

The Western student is apt to be somewhat confused in his ideas regarding the Yogis and their philosophy and practice. Travelers to India have written great tales about the hordes of fakirs, mendicants and mountebanks who infest the great roads of India and the streets of its cities, and who impudently claim the title "Yogi." The Western student is scarcely to be blamed for thinking of the typical Yogi as an emaciated, fanatical, dirty, ignorant Hindu, who either sits in a fixed posture until his body becomes ossified, or else holds his arm up in the air until it becomes stiff and withered and forever after remains in that position, or perhaps clenches his fist and holds it tight until his fingernails grow through the palms of his hands. That these people exist is true, but their claim to the title "Yogi" seems as absurd to the true Yogi as does the claim to the title "Doctor" on the part of the man who parés one's corns seem to the eminent surgeon, or as does the title of "Professor," as assumed by the street corner vendor of worm medicine, seem to the President of Harvard or Yale.

There have been for ages past in India and other Oriental countries men who devoted their time and attention to the development of Man, physically, mentally and spiritually. The experience of generations of earnest seekers has been handed down for centuries from teacher to pupil, and gradually a definite Yogi science was built up. To these investigations and teachings was finally applied the term "Yogi," from the Sanscrit word "Yug," meaning "to join." From the same source comes the English word "yoke," with a similar meaning. Its use in connection with these teachings is difficult to trace, different authorities giving different explanations, but probably the most ingenious is that which holds that it is intended as the Hindu equivalent for the idea conveyed by the English phrase, "getting into harness," or "yoking up," as the Yogi undoubtedly "gets into harness" in his work of controlling the body and mind by the Will.

Yoga is divided into several branches, ranging from that which teaches the control of the body, to that which teaches the attainment of the highest spiritual development. In the work we will not go into the higher phases of the subject, except when the "Science of Breath" touches upon the same. The "Science of Breath" touches Yoga at many points, and although chiefly concerned with the development and control of the physical, has also its psychic side, and even enters the field of spiritual development.

In India there are great schools of Yoga, comprising thousands of the leading minds of that great country. The Yoga philosophy is the rule of life for many people. The pure Yogi teachings, however, are given only to the few, the masses being satisfied with the crumbs which fall from the tables of the educated classes, the Oriental custom in this respect being opposed to that of the Western world. But Western ideas are beginning to have their effect even in the Orient, and teachings which were once given only to the few are now freely offered to any who are ready to receive them. The East and the West are growing closer together, and both are profiting by t..e close contact, each influencing the other.

The Hindu Yogis have always paid great attention to the Science of Breath, for reasons which will be apparent to the student who reads this book. Many Western writers have touched upon this phase of the Yogi teachings, but we believe that it has been reserved for the writer of this work to give to the Western student, in concise form and simple language, the underlying principles of the Yogi Science of Breath, together with many of the favorite Yogi breathing exercises and methods. We have given the Western idea as well as the Oriental, showing how one dovetails into the other. We have used the ordinary English terms, almost entirely, avoiding the Sanscrit terms, so confusing to the average Western reader.

The Yogi practices exercises by which he attains control of his body, and is enabled to send to any organ or part an increased flow of vital force or "prana," thereby strengthening and invigorating the part or organ. He knows all that his Western scientific brother knows about the physiological effect of correct breathing, but he also knows that the air contains more than oxygen and hydrogen and nitrogen, and that something more is accomplished than the mere oxygenating of the blood. He knows something about "prana," of which his Western brother is ignorant, and he is fully aware of the nature and manner of handling that great principle of energy, and is fully informed as to its effect upon the human body and mind. He knows that by rhythmical breathing one may bring himself into harmonious vibration with nature, and aid in the unfoldment of his latent powers. He knows that by controlled breathing he may not only cure disease in himself and others, but also practically do away with fear and worry and the baser emotions.

The Hindu Yogis have always paid great attention to the Science of Breath, for reasons which will be apparent to the student who reads this book. Many Western writers have touched upon this phase of the Yogi teachings, but we believe that it has been reserved for the writer of this work to give to the Western student, in concise form and simple language, the underlying principles of the Yogi Science of Breath, together with many of the favorite Yogi breathing exercises and methods. We have used the ordinary English terms, almost entirely, avoiding the Sanscrit terms, so confusing to the average Western reader.

We may be pardoned if we express ourselves as pleased with our success in condensing so much Yogi lore into so few pages, and by the use of words and terms which may be understood by anyone. Our only fear is that its very simplicity may cause some to pass it by as unworthy of attention, while they pass on their way searching for something "deep," mysterious and non-understandable. However, the Western mind is eminently practical, and we know that it is only a question of a short time before it will recognize the practicability of this work.

Before leaving this part of our subject, however, we wish to say to the reader that he, or she, must not fall into the error of supposing that the knowledge imparted in this little book represents the highest teachings of The Hindu-Yogi philosophers and teachers. On the contrary, the subject of this book is quite elementary, viewed from the standpoint of the advanced Yogi student. Important as are these exercises and information, they belong to the preparatory stage of the work, and their chief value lies in the fact that they enable the student to get his or her body and mind under control, so that the next step may be taken. The Higher Yogi Teachings touch upon and cover many phases. There is "Hatha Yoga," that branch of Yoga which has to do with Physical Well-Being, or Health, and which teaches men and women how to get well and stay well. It might be called Oriental Physical Culture and Hygeine. Then there is "Gnani Yoga" the Yoga of Wisdom, which teaches the deep occult scientific truths underlying the Universe, and Life. Then there is "Raja Yoga," which teaches the Yoga of Mental Development; Will-Power; Thought-Force; Cultivation of the Will; Thought Projection; Mental Influence, etc., etc. These, and other branches of Yoga, form the subject of a series of books being issued by the publishers of this little book, full notice of which may be seen by reference to the pages following the exercises, etc.

CHAPTER II.
THE SECRET OF PRANA.

The Science of Breath, like many other teachings, has its esoteric or inner phase, as well as its exoteric or external. The physiological phase may be termed the outer or exoteric side of the subject, and the phase which we will now consider may be termed its esoteric or inner side. Occultists, in all ages and lands, have always taught, usually secretly to a few followers, that there was to be found in the air a substance or principle from which all activity, vitality and life was derived. They differed in their terms and names for this force, as well as in the details of the theory, but the main principle is to be found in all occult teachings and philosophies, and has for centuries formed a portion of the teachings of the Oriental Yogis.

In order to avoid misconceptions arising from the various theories regarding this great principle, which theories are usually attached to some name given the principle, we, in this work, will speak of the principle as "Prana," this word being the Sanscrit term meaning "Absolute Energy." Many occult authorities teach that the principle which the Hindus term "Prana" is the universal principle of energy or force, and that all energy or force is derived from that principle, or, rather, is a particular form of manifestation of that principle. These theories do not concern us in the consideration of the subject matter of this work, and we will therefore confine ourselves to an understanding of prana as the principle of energy exhibited in all living things, which distinguishes them from a lifeless thing. We may consider it as the active principle of life—Vital Force, if you please. It is found in all forms of life, from the amoeba to man—from the most elementary form of plant life to the highest form of animal life. Prana is all pervading. It is found in all things having life, and as the occult philosophy teaches that life is in all things—in every atom—the apparent lifelessness of some things being only a lesser degree of manifestation, we may understand their teachings that prana is everywhere, in everything. Prana must not be confounded with the Ego—that bit of Divine Spirit in every soul, around which clusters matter and energy. Prana is merely a form of energy used by the Ego in its material manifestation. When the Ego leaves the body, the prana, being no longer under its control, responds only to the orders of the individual atoms, or groups of atoms, forming the body, and as the body disintegrates and is resolved to its original elements, each atom takes with it sufficient prana to enable it to form new combinations, the unused prana returning to the great universal storehouse from which it came. With the Ego in control, cohesion exists and the atoms are held together by the Will of the Ego.

Prana is the name by which we designate a universal principle, which principle is the essence of all motion, force or energy, whether manifested in gravitation, electricity, the revolution of the planets, and all forms of life, from the highest to the lowest. It may be called the soul of Force and Energy in all their forms, and that principle which, operating in a certain way, causes that form of activity which accompanies Life.

This great principle is in all forms of matter, and yet it is not matter. It is in the air, but it is not the air nor one of its chemical constituents. Animal and plant life breathe it in with the air, and yet if the air contained it not they would die even though they might be filled with air. It is taken up by the system along with the oxygen, and yet is not the oxygen. The Hebrew writer of the book of Genesis knew the difference between the atmospheric air and the mysterious and potent principle contained within it. He speaks of neshemet ruach chayim, which, translated, means "the breath of the spirit of life." In the Hebrew neshemet means the ordinary breath of atmospheric air, and chayim means life or lives, while the word ruach means the "spirit of life," which occultists claim is the same principle which we speak of as Prana.

Prana is in the atmospheric air, but it is also elsewhere, and it penetrates where the air cannot reach. The oxygen in the air plays an important part in sustaining animal life, and the carbon plays a similar part with plant life, but Prana has its own distinct part to play in the manifestation of life, aside from the physiological functions.

We are constantly inhaling the air charged with prana, and are as constantly extracting the latter from the air and appropriating it to our uses. Prana is found in its freest state in the atmospheric air, which when fresh is fairly charged with it, and we draw it to us more easily from the air than from any other source. In ordinary breathing we absorb and extract a normal supply of prana, but by controlled and regulated breathing (generally known as Yogi breathing) we are enabled to extract a greater supply, which is stored away in the brain and nerve centers, to be used when necessary. We may store away prana, just as the storage battery stores away electricity. The many powers attributed to advanced occultists is due largely to their knowledge of this fact and their intelligent use of this stored-up energy. The Yogis know that by certain forms of breathing they establish certain relations with the supply of prana and may draw on the same for what they require. Not only do they strengthen all parts of their body in this way, but the brain itself may receive increased energy from the same source, and latent faculties be developed and psychic powers attained. One who has mastered the science of storing away prana, either consciously or unconsciously, often radiates vitality and strength which is felt by those coming in contact with him, and such a person may impart this strength to others, and give them increased vitality and health. What is called "magnetic healing" is performed in this way, although many practitioners are not aware of the source of their power.

Western scientists have been dimly aware of this great principle with which the air is charged, but finding that they could find no chemical trace of it, or make it register on any of their instruments, they have generally treated the Oriental theory with disdain. They could not explain this principle, and so denied it. They seem, however, to recognize that the air in certain places possesses a greater amount of "something" and sick people are directed by their physicians to seek such places in hopes of regaining lost health.

The oxygen in the air is appropriated by the blood and is made use of by the circulatory system. The prana in the air is appropriated by the nervous system, and is used in its work. And as the oxygenated blood is carried to all parts of the system, building up and replenishing, so is the prana carried to all parts of the nervous system, adding strength and vitality. If we think of prana as being the active principle of what we call "vitality," we will be able to form a much clearer idea of what an important part it plays in our lives. Just as is the oxygen in the blood used up by the wants of the system, so the supply of prana taken up by the nervous system is exhausted by our thinking, willing, acting, etc., and in consequence constant replenishing is necessary. Every thought, every act, every effort of the will, every motion of a muscle, uses up a certain amount of what we call nerve force, which is really a form of prana. To move a muscle the brain sends out an impulse over the nerves, and the muscle contracts, and so much prana is expended. When it is remembered that the greater portion of prana acquired by man comes to him from the air inhaled, the importance of proper breathing is readily understood.

CHAPTER III

THE YOGI COMPLETE BREATH.

The Yogi Complete Breath is the fundamental breath of the entire Yogi Science of Breath, and the student must fully acquaint himself with it, and master it perfectly before he can hope to obtain results from the other forms of breath mentioned and given in this book. He should not be content with half-learning it, but should go to work in earnest until it becomes his natural method of breathing. This will require work, time and patience, but without these things nothing is ever accomplished. There is no royal road to the Science of Breath, and the student must be prepared to practice and study in earnest if he expect to receive results. The results obtained by a complete mastery of the Science of Breath are great, and no one who has attained them would willingly go back to the old methods, and he will tell his friends that he considers himself amply repaid for all his work. We say these things now, that you may fully understand the necessity and importance of mastering this fundamental method of Yogi Breathing, instead of passing it by and trying some of the attractive looking variations given later on in this book. Again, we say to you: Start right, and right results will follow; but neglect your foundations and your entire building will topple over sooner or later.

Perhaps the better way to teach you how to develop the Yogi Complete Breath, would be to give you simple directions regarding the breath itself, and then follow up the same with general remarks concerning it, and then later on giving exercises for developing the chest, muscles and lungs which have been allowed to remain in an undeveloped condition by imperfect methods of breathing. Right here we wish to say that this Complete Breath is not a forced or abnormal thing, but on the contrary is a going back to first principles—a return to Nature. The healthy adult savage and the healthy infant of civilization both breathe in this manner, but civilized man has adopted

unnatural methods of living, clothing, etc., and has lost
his birthright. And we wish to remind the reader that
the Complete Breath does not necessarily call for the complete filling of the lungs at every inhalation. One may
inhale the average amount of air, using the Complete
Breathing Method and distributing the air inhaled, be the
quantity large or small, to all parts of the lungs. But one
should inhale a series of full Complete Breaths several
times a day, whenever opportunity offers, in order to keep
the system in good order and condition.

The following simple exercise will give you a clear
idea of what the Complete Breath is:

(1) Stand or sit erect. Breathing through the nostrils, inhale steadily, first filling the lower part of the
lungs, which is accomplished by bringing into play the
diaphragm, which descending exerts a gentle pressure on
the abdominal organs, pushing forward the front walls of
the abdomen. Then fill the middle part of the lungs, pushing out the lower ribs, breast-bone and chest. Then fill
the higher portion of the lungs, protruding the upper chest,
thus lifting the chest, including the upper six or seven
pairs of ribs. In the final movement, the lower part of
the abdomen will be slightly drawn in, which movement
gives the lungs a support and also helps to fill the highest
part of the lungs.

At first reading it may appear that this breath consists
of three distinct movements. This, however, is not the
correct idea. The inhalation is continuous, the entire chest
cavity from the lowered diaphragm to the highest point
of the chest in the region of the collar-bone, being expanded
with a uniform movement. Avoid a jerky series of inhalations, and strive to attain a steady continuous action. Practice will soon overcome the tendency to divide the inhalation into three movements, and will result in a uniform continuous breath. You will be able to complete the inhalation in a couple of seconds after a little practice.

(2) Retain the breath a few seconds.

(3) Exhale quite slowly, holding the chest in a firm
position, and drawing the abdomen in a little and lifting it
upward slowly as the air leaves the lungs. When the air is

entirely exhaled, relax the chest and abdomen. A little practice will render this part of the exercise easy, and the movement once acquired will be afterwards performed almost automatically.

It will be seen that by this method of breathing all parts of the respiratory apparatus is brought into action, and all parts of the lungs, including the most remote air cells, are exercised. The chest cavity is expanded in all directions. You will also notice that the Complete Breath is really a combination of Low, Mid and High Breaths, succeeding each other rapidly in the order given, in such a manner as to form one uniform, continuous, complete breath.

You will find it quite a help to you if you will practice this breath before a large mirror, placing the hands lightly over the abdomen so that you may feel the movements. At the end of the inhalation, it is well to occasionally slightly elevate the shoulders, thus raising the collarbone and allowing the air to pass freely into the small upper lobe of the right lung, which place is sometimes the breeding place of tuberculosis.

At the beginning of practice, you may have more or less trouble in acquiring the Complete Breath, but a little practice will make perfect, and when you have once acquired it you will never willingly return to the old methods.

CHAPTER IV.

A FEW BITS OF YOGI LORE.

We give below three forms of breath, quite popular among the Yogis. The first is the well-known Yogi Cleansing Breath, to which is attributed much of the great lung endurance found among the Yogis. They usually finish up a breathing exercise with this Cleansing Breath, and we have followed this plan in this book. We also give the Yogi Nerve Vitalizing Exercise, which has been handed down among them for ages, and which has never been improved on by Western teachers of Physical Culture, although some of them have "borrowed" it from teachers of Yoga. We also give the Yogi Vocal Breath, which accounts largely for the melodious, vibrant voices of the better class of the Oriental Yogis. We feel that if this book contained nothing more than these three exercises, it would be invaluable to the Western student. Take these exercises as a gift from your Eastern brothers and put them into practice.

THE YOGI CLEANSING BREATH.

The Yogis have a favorite form of breathing which they practice when they feel the necessity of ventilating and cleansing the lungs. They conclude many of their other breathing exercises with this breath, and we have followed this practice in this book. This Cleansing Breath ventilates and cleanses the lungs, stimulates the cells and gives a general tone to the respiratory organs, and is conducive to their general healthy condition. Besides this effect, it is found to greatly refresh the entire system. Speakers, singers, etc., will find this breath especially restful, after having tired the respiratory organs.

(1) Inhale a complete breath.

(2) Retain the air a few seconds.

(3) Pucker up the lips as if for a whistle (but do not swell out the cheeks), then exhale a little air through the opening, with considerable vigor. Then stop for a moment,

16

retaining the air, and then exhale a little more **air.** Repeat until the air is completely exhaled. Remember that considerable vigor is to be used in exhaling the air through the opening in the lips.

This breath will be found quite refreshing when one is tired and generally "used up." A trial will convince the student of its merits. This exercise should be practiced until it can be performed naturally and easily, as it is used to finish up a number of other exercises given in this book, and it should be thoroughly understood.

THE YOGI NERVE VITALIZING BREATH.

This is an exercise well known to the Yogis, who consider it one of the strongest nerve stimulants and invigorants known to man. Its purpose is to stimulate the Nervous System, develop nerve force, energy and vitality. This exercise brings a stimulating pressure to bear on important nerve centers, which in turn stimulate and energize the entire nervous system, and send an increased flow of nerve force to all parts of the body.

(1) Stand erect.

(2) Inhale a Complete Breath, and retain same.

(3) Extend the arms straight in front of you, letting them be somewhat limp and relaxed, with only sufficient nerve force to hold them out.

(4) Slowly draw the hands back toward the shoulders, gradually contracting the muscles and putting force into them, so that when they reach the shoulders the fists will be so tightly clenched that a tremulous motion is felt.

(5) Then, keeping the muscles tense, push the fists slowly out, and then draw them back rapidly (still tense) several times.

(6) Exhale vigorously through the mouth.

(7) Practice the Cleansing Breath.

The efficiency of this exercise depends greatly upon the speed of the drawing back of the fists, and the tension of the muscles, and, of course, upon the full lungs. This exercise must be tried to be appreciated. It is without equal as a "bracer," as our Western friends put it.

THE YOGI VOCAL BREATH.

The Yogis have a form of breathing to develop the voice. They are noted for their wonderful voices, which are strong, smooth and clear, and have a wonderful trumpet-like carrying power. They have practiced this particular form of breathing exercise which has resulted in rendering their voices soft, beautiful and flexible, imparting to it that indescribable, peculiar floating quality, combined with great power. The exercise given below will in time impart the above-mentioned qualities, or the Yogi Voice, to the student who practices it faithfully. It is to be understood, of course, that this form of breath is to be used only as an occasional exercise, and not as a regular form of breathing.

(1) Inhale a Complete Breath very slowly, but steadily, through the nostrils, taking as much time as possible in the inhalation.

(2) Retain for a few seconds.

(3) Expel the air vigorously in one great breath, through the wide opened mouth.

(4) Rest the lungs by the Cleansing Breath.

Without going deeply into the Yogi theories of sound-production in speaking and singing, we wish to say that experience has taught them that the timbre, quality and power of a voice depends not alone upon the vocal organs in the throat, but that the facial muscles, etc., have much to do with the matter. Some men with large chests produce but a poor tone, while others with comparatively small chests produce tones of amazing strength and quality. Here is an interesting experiment worth trying: Stand before a glass and pucker up your mouth and whistle, and note the shape of your mouth and the general expression of your face. Then sing or speak as you do naturally, and see the difference. Then start to whistle again for a few seconds, and then, *without changing the position of your lips or face*, sing a few notes and notice what a vibrant, resonant, clear and beautiful tone is produced.

CHAPTER V.

THE SEVEN YOGI DEVELOPING EXERCISES.

The following are the seven favorite exercises of the Yogis for developing the lungs, muscles, ligaments, air cells, etc. They are quite simple but marvelously effective. Do not let the simplicity of these exercises make you lose interest, for they are the result of careful experiments and practice on the part of the Yogis, and are the essence of numerous intricate and complicated exercises, the non-essential portions being eliminated and the essential features retained.

(1) THE RETAINED BREATH.

This is a very important exercise which tends to strengthen and develop the respiratory muscles as well as the lungs, and its frequent practice will also tend to expand the chest. The Yogis have found that an occasional holding of the breath, after the lungs have been filled with the Complete Breath, is very beneficial, not only to the respiratory organs but to the organs of nutrition, the nervous system and the blood itself. They have found that an occasional holding of the breath tends to purify the air which has remained in the lungs from former inhalations, and to more fully oxygenate the blood. They also know that the breath so retained gathers up all the waste matter, and when the breath is expelled it carries with it the effete matter of the system, and cleanses the lungs just as a purgative does the bowels. The Yogis recommend this exercise for various disorders of the stomach, liver and blood, and also find that it frequently relieves bad breath, which often arises from poorly ventilated lungs. We recommend students to pay considerable attention to this exercise, as it has great merits. The following directions will give you a clear idea of the exercise:

(1) Stand erect.

(2) Inhale a Complete Breath.

(3) Retain the air as long as you can comfortably.

19

(4) Exhale vigorously through the open mouth.

(5) Practice the Cleansing Breath.

At first you will be able to retain the breath only a short time, but a little practice will also show a great improvement. Time yourself with a watch if you wish to note your progress.

(2) LUNG CELL STIMULATION.

This exercise is designed to stimulate the air cells in the lungs, but beginners must not overdo it, and in no case should it be indulged in too vigorously. Some may find a slight dizziness resulting from the first few trials, in which case let them walk around a little and discontinue the exercise for a while.

(1) Stand erect, with hands at sides.

(2) Breathe in very slowly and gradually.

(3) While inhaling, gently tap the chest with the finger tips, constantly changing position.

(4) When the lungs are filled, retain the breath and pat the chest with the palms of the hands.

(5) Practice the Cleansing Breath.

This exercise is very bracing and stimulating to the whole body, and is a well-known Yogi practice. Many of the air cells of the lungs become inactive by reason of incomplete breathing, and often become almost atrophied. One who has practiced imperfect breathing for years will find it not so easy to stimulate all these ill-used air cells into activity all at once by the Complete Breath, but this exercise will do much toward bringing about the desired result, and is worth study and practice.

(3) RIB STRETCHING.

We have explained that the ribs are fastened by cartilages, which admit of considerable expansion. In proper breathing, the ribs play an important part, and it is well to occasionally give them a little special exercise in order to preserve their elasticity. Standing or sitting in unnatural positions, to which many of the Western people are addicted, is apt to render the ribs more or less stiff and inelastic, and this exercise will do much to overcome same.

(1) Stand erect.

(2) Place the hands one on each side of the body, as high up under the armpits as convenient, the thumbs reaching toward the back, the palms on the side of the chest and the fingers to the front over the breast.

(3) Inhale a Complete Breath.

(4) Retain the air for a short time.

(5) Then gently squeeze the sides, at the same time slowly exhaling.

(6) Practice the cleansing breath.

Use moderation in this exercise and do not overdo it

(4) CHEST EXPANSION.

The chest is quite apt to be contracted from bending over one's work, etc. This exercise is very good for the purpose of restoring natural conditions and gaining chest expansion.

(1) Stand erect.

(2) Inhale a Complete Breath.

(3) Retain the air.

(4) Extend both arms forward and bring the two clenched fists together on a level with the shoulder.

(5) Then swing back the fists vigorously until the arms stand out straight sideways from the shoulders.

(6) Then bring back to Position 4, and swing to Position 5. Repeat several times.

(7) Exhale vigorously through the opened mouth.

(8) Practice the Cleansing Breath.

Use moderation and do not overdo this exercise.

(5) WALKING EXERCISE.

(1) Walk with head up, chin drawn slightly in, shoulders back, and with measured tread.

(2) Inhale a Complete Breath, counting (mentally) 1, 2, 3, 4, 5, 6, 7, 8, one count to each step, making the inhalation extend over the eight counts.

(3) Exhale slowly through the nostrils, counting as before—1, 2, 3, 4, 5, 6, 7, 8—one count to a step.

(4) Rest between breaths, continuing walking and counting, 1, 2, 3, 4, 5, 6, 7, 8, one count to a step.

(5) Repeat until you begin to feel tired. Then rest for a while, and resume at pleasure. Repeat several times a day.

Some Yogis vary this exercise by retaining the breath during a 1, 2, 3, 4, count, and then exhale in an eight-step count. Practice whichever plan seems most agreeable to you.

(6) MORNING EXERCISE.

(1) Stand erect in a military attitude, head up, eyes front, shoulders back, knees stiff, hands at sides.

(2) Raise body slowly on toes, inhaling a Complete Breath, steadily and slowly.

(3) Retain the breath for a few seconds, maintaining the same position.

(4) Slowly sink to first position, at the same time slowly exhaling the air through the nostrils.

(5) Practice Cleansing Breath.

(6) Repeat several times, varying by using right leg alone, then left leg alone.

(7) STIMULATING CIRCULATION.

(1) Stand erect.

(2) Inhale a Complete Breath and retain.

(3) Bend forward slightly and grasp a stick or cane steadily and firmly, and gradually exerting your entire strength upon the grasp.

(4) Relax the grasp, return to first position, and slowly exhale.

(5) Repeat several times.

(6) Finish with the Cleansing Breath.

This exercise may be performed without the use of a stick or cane, by grasping an imaginary cane, using the will to exert the pressure. The exercise is a favorite Yogi plan of stimulating the circulation by driving the arterial blood to the extremities, and drawing back the venous blood to the heart and lungs that it may take up the oxygen which has been inhaled with the air.

CHAPTER VI.
SEVEN MINOR YOGI EXERCISES.

This chapter is composed of seven minor Yogi Breathing Exercises, bearing no special names, but each distinct and separate from the others and having a different purpose in view. Each student will find several of these exercises best adapted to the special requirements of his particular case. Although we have styled these exercises "minor exercises," they are quite valuable and useful, or they would not appear in this book. They give one a condensed course in "Physical Culture" and "Lung Development," and might readily be "padded out" and elaborated into a small book on these subjects. They have, of course, an additional value, as Yogi Breathing forms a part of each exercise. Do not pass them by becaue they are marked "minor." Some one or more of these exercises may be just what you need. Try them and decide for yourself.

EXERCISE I.

(1) Stand erect with hands at sides.

(2) Inhale Complete Breath.

(3) Raise the arms slowly, keeping them rigid until the hands touch over head.

(4) Retain the breath a few minutes with hands over head.

(5) Lower hands slowly to sides, exhaling slowly at same time.

(6) Practice Cleansing Breath.

EXERCISE II.

(1) Stand erect, with arms straight in front of you.

(2) Inhale Complete Breath and retain.

(3) Swing arms back as far as they will go; then back to first position; then repeat several times, retaining the breath all the while.

(4) Exhale vigorously through mouth.

(5) Practice Cleansing Breath.

EXERCISE III.

(1) Stand erect with arms straight in front of you.

(2) Inhale Complete Breath.

(3) Swing arms around in a circle, backward, a few times. Then reverse a few times, retaining the breath all the while. You may vary this by rotating them alternately like the sails of a windmill.

(4) Exhale the breath vigorously through the mouth.

(5) Practice Cleansing Breath.

EXERCISE IV.

(1) Lie on the floor with your face downward and palms of hands flat upon the floor by your sides.

(2) Inhale Complete Breath and retain.

(3) Stiffen the body and raise yourself up by the strength of your arms until you rest on your hands and toes

(4) Then lower yourself to original position. Repeat several times.

(5) Exhale vigorously through your mouth.

(6) Practice Cleansing Breath.

EXERCISE V.

(1) Stand erect with your palms against the wall.

(2) Inhale Complete Breath and retain.

(3) Lower the chest to the wall, resting your weight on your hands.

(4) Then raise yourself back with the arm muscles alone, keeping the body stiff.

(5) Exhale vigorously through the mouth.

(6) Practice Cleansing Breath.

EXERCISE VI.

(1) Stand erect with arms "akimbo," that is, with hands resting around the waist and elbows standing out.

(2) Inhale Complete Breath and retain.

(3) Keep legs and hips stiff and bend well forward, as if bowing, at the same time exhaling slowly.

(4) Return to first position and take another Complete Breath.

(5) Then bend backward, exhaling slowly.

(6) Return to first position and take a Complete Breath.

(7) Then bend sideways, exhaling slowly. (Vary by bending to right and then to left.)

(8) Practice Cleansing Breath.

EXERCISE VII.

(1) Stand erect, or sit erect, with straight spinal column.

(2) Inhale a Complete Breath, but instead of inhaling in a continuous steady stream, take a series of short, quick "sniffs," as if you were smelling aromatic salts or ammonia and did not wish to get too strong a "whiff." Do not exhale any of these little breaths, but add one to the other until the entire lung space is filled.

(3) Retain for a few seconds.

(4) Exhale through the nostrils in a long, restful, sighing breath.

(5) Practice Cleansing Breath.

CHAPTER VII.

VIBRATION AND YOGI RHYTHMIC BREATHING

All is in vibration. From the tiniest atom to the greatest sun, everything is in a state of vibration. There is nothing in absolute rest in nature. A single atom deprived of vibration would wreck the universe. In incessant vibration the universal work is performed. Matter is being constantly played upon by energy and countless forms and numberless varieties result, and yet even the forms and varieties are not permanent. They begin to change the moment they are created, and from them are born innumerable forms, which in turn change and give rise to newer forms, and so on and on, in infinite succession. Nothing is permanent in the world of forms, and yet the great Reality is unchangeable. Forms are but appearances—they come, they go, but the Reality is eternal and unchangeable.

The atoms of the human body are in constant vibration. Unceasing changes are occurring. In a few months there is almost a complete change in the matter composing the body, and scarcely a single atom now composing your body will be found in it a few months hence. Vibration, constant vibration. Change, constant change.

In all vibration is to be found a certain rhythm. Rhythm pervades the universe. The swing of the planets around the sun; the rise and fall of the sea; the beating of the heart; the ebb and flow of the tide; all follow rhythmic laws. The rays of the sun reach us; the rain descends upon us, in obedience to the same law. All growth is but an exhibition of this law. All motion is a manifestation of the law of rhythm.

Our bodies are as much subject to rhythmic laws as is the planet in its revolution around the sun. Much of the esoteric side of the Yogi Science of Breath is based upon this known principle of nature. By falling in with the rhythm of the body, the Yogi manages to absorb a great amount of Prana, which he disposes of to bring about

26

results desired by him. We will speak of this at greater length later on.

The body which you occupy is like a small inlet running in to the land from the sea. Although apparently subject only to its own laws, it is really subject to the ebb and flow of the tides of the ocean. The great sea of life is swelling and receding, rising and falling, and we are responding to its vibrations and rhythm. In a normal condition we receive the vibration and rhythm of the great ocean of life, and respond to it, but at times the mouth of the inlet seems choked up with debris, and we fail to receive the impulse from Mother Ocean, and inharmony manifests within us.

You have heard how a note on a violin, if sounded repeatedly and in rhythm, will start into motion vibrations which will in time destroy a bridge. The same result is true when a regiment of soldiers crosses a bridge, the order being always given to "break step" on such an occasion, lest the vibration bring down both bridge and regiment. These manifestations of the effect of rhythmic motion will give you an idea of the effect on the body of rhythmic breathing. The whole system catches the vibration and becomes in harmony with the will, which causes the rhythmic motion of the lungs, and while in such complete harmony will respond readily to orders from the will. With the body thus attuned, the Yogi finds no difficulty in increasing the circulation in any part of the body by an order from the will, and in the same way he can direct an increased current of nerve force to any part or organ, strengthening and stimulating it.

In the same way the Yogi by rhythmic breathing "catches the swing," as it were, and is able to absorb and control a greatly increased amount of prana, which is then at the disposal of his will. He can and does use it as a vehicle for sending forth thoughts to others and for attracting to him all those whose thoughts are keyed in the same vibration. The phenomena of telepathy, thought transference, mental healing, mesmerism, etc., which subjects are creating such an interest in the Western world at the present time, but which have been known to the

Yogis for centuries, can be greatly increased and augmented if the person sending forth the thoughts will do so after rhythmic breathing. Rhythmic breathing will increase the value of mental healing, magnetic healing, etc., several hundred per cent.

In rhythmic breathing the main thing to be acquired is the mental idea of rhythm. To those who know anything of music, the idea of measured counting is familiar. To others, the rhythmic step of the soldier: "Left, right; left, right; left, right; one, two, three, four; one, two, three, four," will convey the idea.

The Yogi bases his rhythmic time upon a unit corresponding with the beat of his heart. The heart beat varies in different persons, but the heart beat unit of each person is the proper rhythmic standard for that particular individual in his rhythmic breathing. Ascertain your normal heart beat by placing your fingers over your pulse, and then count: "1, 2, 3, 4, 5, 6; 1, 2, 3, 4, 5, 6," etc., until the rhythm becomes firmly fixed in your mind. A little practice will fix the rhythm, so that you will be able to easily reproduce it. The beginner usually inhales in about six pulse units, but he will be able to greatly increase this by practice.

The Yogi rule for rhythmic breathing is that the units of inhalation and exhalation should be the same, while the units for retention and between breaths should be one-half the number of those of inhalation and exhalation.

The following exercise in Rhythmic Breathing should be thoroughly mastered, as it forms the basis of numerous other exercises, to which reference will be made later.

(1) Sit erect, in an easy posture, being sure to hold the chest, neck and head as nearly in a straight line as possible, with shoulders slightly thrown back and hands resting easily on the lap. In this position the weight of the body is largely supported by the ribs and the position may be easily maintained. The Yogi has found that one cannot get the best effect of rhythmic breathing with the chest drawn in and the abdomen protruding.

(2) Inhale slowly a Complete Breath, counting six pulse units.

(3) Retain, counting three pulse units.

(4) Exhale slowly through the nostrils, counting six pulse units.

(5) Count three pulse beats between breaths.

(6) Repeat a number of times, but avoid fatiguing yourself at the start.

(7) When you are ready to close the exercise, practice the cleansing breath, which will rest you and cleanse the lungs.

After a little practice you will be able to increase the duration of the inhalations and exhalations, until about fifteen pulse units are consumed. In this increase, remember that the units for retention and between breaths is one-half the units for inhalation and exhalation.

Do not overdo yourself in your effort to increase the duration of the breath, but pay as much attention as possible to acquiring the "rhythm," as that is more important than the length of the breath. Practice and try until you get the measured "swing" of the movement, and until you can almost "feel" the rhythm of the vibratory motion throughout your whole body. It will require a little practice and perseverance, but your pleasure at your improvement will make the task an easy one. The Yogi is a most patient and persevering man, and his great attainments are due largely to the possession of these qualities.

CHAPTER VIII.
YOGI PSYCHIC BREATHING.

With the exception of the instructions in the **Yogi Rhythmic Breathing**, the majority of the exercises heretofore given in this book relate to the physical plane of effort, which, while highly important in itself, is also regarded by the Yogis as in the nature of affording a sub stantial basis for efforts on the psychic and spiritual plane Do not, however, discard or think lightly of the physical phase of the subject, for remember that it needs a sound body to support a sound mind, and also that the body is the temple of the Ego, the lamp in which burns the light of the Spirit. Everything is good in its place, and everything has its place. The developed man is the "all-around man," who recognizes body, mind and spirit and renders to each its due. Neglect of either is a mistake which must be rectified sooner or later; a debt which must be repaid with interest.

We will now take up the Psychic phase of the Yogi Science of Breath in the shape of a series of exercises, each exercise carrying with it its explanation.

You will notice that in each exercise rhythmic breathing is accompanied with the instructions to "carry the thought" of certain desired results. This mental attitude gives the Will a cleared track upon which to exercise its force. We cannot, in this work, go into the subject of the power of the Will, and must assume that you have some knowledge of the subject. If you have no acquaintance with the subject, you will find that the actual practice of the exercises themselves will give you a much clearer knowledge than any amount of theoretical teaching, for as the old Hindu proverb says, "He who tastes a grain of mustard seed knows more of its flavor than he who sees an elephant load of it."

(1) GENERAL DIRECTIONS FOR YOGI PSYCHIC BREATHING.

The basis of all Yogi Psychic Breathing is the **Yogi Rhythmic Breath**, instruction regarding which we gave in our last chapter. In the following exercises, in order to avoid useless repetition, we will say merely, "Breathe Rhythmically," and then give the instruction for the exercise of the psychic force, or directed Will power working in connection with the rhythmic breath vibrations. After a little practice you will find that you will not need to count after the first rhythmic breath, as the mind will grasp the idea of time and rhythm and you will be able to breathe rhythmically at pleasure, almost automatically. This will leave the mind clear for the sending of the psychic vibrations under the direction of the Will. (See the following first exercise for directions in using the Will.)

(2) PRANA DISTRIBUTING.

Lying flat on the floor or bed, completely relaxed, with hands resting lightly over the Solar Plexus (over the pit of the stomach, where the ribs begin to separate), breathe rhythmically. After the rhythm is fully establshed *will* that each inhalation will draw in an increased supply of prana or vital energy from the Universal supply, which will be taken up by the nervous system and stored in the Solar Plexus. At each exhalation will that the prana or vital energy is being distributed all over the body, to every organ and part; to every muscle, cell and atom; to nerve, artery and vein; from the top of your head to the soles of your feet; invigorating, strengthening and stimulating every nerve; recharging every nerve center; sending energy, force and strength all over the system. While exercising the will, try to form a mental picture of the inrushing prana, coming in through the lungs and being taken up at once by the Solar Plexus, then with the exhaling effort, being sent to all parts of the system, down to the finger tips and down to the toes. It is not necessary to use the Will with an effort. Simply commanding that which you wish to produce and then making the mental picture of it is all that is necessary. Calm command with the mental picture is far better than forcible willing, which only dissipates force needlessly. The above exercise is most helpful and greatly refreshes and strengthens the nervous system and produces a restful feeling all over the body. It is especially beneficial in cases where one is tired or feels a lack of energy.

(3) INHIBITING PAIN.

Lying down or sitting erect, breath rhythmically, holding the thought that you are inhaling prana. Then when you exhale, send the prana to the painful part to re-establish the circulation and nerve current. Then inhale more prana for the purpose of driving out the painful condition; then exhale, holding the thought that you are driving out the pain. Alternate the two above mental commands, and with one exhalation stimulate the part and with the next drive out the pain. Keep this up for seven breaths, then practice the Cleansing Breath and rest a while. Then try it again until relief comes, which will be before long. Many pains will be found to be relieved before the seven breaths are finished. If the hand is placed over the painful part, you may get quicker results. Send the current of prana down the arm and into the painful part.

(4) DIRECTING THE CIRCULATION.

Lying down or sitting erect, breathe rhythmically, and with the exhalations direct the circulation to any part you wish, which may be suffering from imperfect circulation. This is effective in cases of cold feet or in cases of headache, the blood being sent downward in both cases, in the first case warming the feet, and in the latter, relieving the brain from too great pressure. In the case of headache, try the Pain Inhibiting first, then follow with sending the blood downward. You will often feel a warm feeling in the legs as the circulation moves downward. The circulation is largely under the control of the will and rhythmic breathing renders the task easier.

(5) SELF-HEALING.

Lying in a relaxed condition, breathe rhythmically, and command that a good supply of prana be inhaled. With the exhalation, send the prana to the affected part for the purpose of stimulating it. Vary this occasionally by exhaling, with the mental command that the diseased condition be forced out and disappear. Use the hands in this exercise, passing them down the body from the head to the affected part. In using the hands in healing yourself or others always hold the mental image that the prana is flowing down the arm and through the finger tips into the body, thus reaching the affected part and healing it. Of course we can give only general directions in this book without taking up the several forms of disease in detail, but a little practice of the above exercise, varying it slightly to fit the conditions of the case, will produce wonderful results. Some Yogis follow the plan of placing both hands on the affected part, and then breathing rhythmically, holding the mental image that they are fairly pumping prana into the diseased organ and part, stimulating it and driving out diseased conditions, as pumping into a pail of dirty water will drive out the latter and fill the bucket with fresh water. This last plan is very effective if the mental image of the pump is clearly held, the inhalation representing the lifting of the pump handle and the exhalation the actual pumping.

(6) HEALING OTHERS.

We cannot take up the question of the psychic treatment of disease by prana in detail in this book, as such would be foreign to its purpose. But we can and will give you simple, plain instructions whereby you may be enabled to do much good in relieving others. The main principle to remember is that by rhythmic breathing and controlled thought you are enabled to absorb a considerable amount of prana, and are also able to pass it into the body of another person, stimulating weakened parts and organs and imparting health and driving out diseased conditions. You must first learn to form such a clear mental image of the desired condition that you will be able to actually feel the influx of prana, and the force running down your arms and out of your finger tips into the body of the patient. Breathe rhythmically a few times until the rhythm is fairly established, then place your hands upon the affected part of the body of the patient, letting them rest lightly over the part. Then follow the "pumping" process described in the preceding exercise (Self-Healing) and fill the patient full of prana until the diseased condition is driven out. Every once in a while raise the hands and "flick" the fingers as if you were throwing off the diseased condition. It is well to do this occasionally and also to wash the hands after treatment, as otherwise you may take on a trace of the diseased condition of the patient. Also practice the Cleansing Breath several times after the treatment. During the treatment let the prana pour into the patient in one continuous stream, allowing yourself to be merely the pumping machinery connecting the patient with the universal supply of prana, and allowing it to flow freely through you. You need not work the hands vigorously, but simply enough that the prana freely reaches the affected parts. The rhythmic breathing must be practiced frequently during the treatment, so as to keep the rhythm normal and to afford the prana a free passage. It is better to place the hands on the bare skin, but where this is not advisable or possible place them over the clothing. Vary above method occasionally during the treatment by stroking the body gently and softly with the finger tips, the fingers being kept slightly separated. This is very soothing to the patient. In cases of long standing you may find it helpful to give the mental command in words, such as "get out, get out," or "be strong, be strong," as the case may be, the words helping you to exercise the will more forcibly and to the point. Vary these instructions to suit the needs of the case, and use your own judgment and inventive faculty. We have given you the general principles and you can apply them in hundreds of different ways. The above apparently simple instruction, if carefully studied and applied, will enable one to accomplish all that the leading "magnetic healers" are able to, although their "systems" are more or less cumbersome and complicated. They are using prana ignorantly and calling it "magnetism." If they would combine rhythmic breathing with their "magnetic" treatment they would double their efficiency.

(7) DISTANT HEALING.

Prana colored by the thought of the sender may be projected to persons at a distance, who are willing to re-

ceive it, and healing work done in this way. This is the
secret of the "absent healing," of which the Western world
has heard so much of late years. The thought of the healer
sends forth and colors the prana of the sender, and it
flashes across space and finds lodgment in the psychic mechanism of the patient. It is unseen, and like the Marconi
waves, it passes through intervening obstacles and seeks
the person attuned to receive it. In order to treat persons
at a distance, you must form a mental image of them until
you can feel yourself to be en rapport with them. This is
a psychic process dependent upon the mental imagery
of the healer. You can feel the sense of rapport when it
is established, it manifesting in a sense of nearness. That
is about as plain as we can describe it. It may be acquired
by a little practice, and some will get it at the first trial.
When rapport is established, say mentally to the distant
patient, "I am sending you a supply of vital force or power,
which will invigorate you and heal you." Then picture
the prana as leaving your mind with each exhalation of
rhythmic breath, and traveling across space instantaneously
and reaching the patient and healing him. It is not necessary to fix certain hours for treatment, although you may
do so if you wish. The receptive condition of the patient,
as he is expecting and opening himself up to your psychic
force, attunes him to receive your vibrations whenever you
may send them. If you agree upon hours, let him place
himself in a relaxed attitude and receptive condition. The
above is the great underlying principle of the "absent treatment" of the Western world. You may do these things as
well as the most noted healers, with a little practice.

CHAPTER IX.
THOUGHT-FORCE, ETC.

(1) THOUGHT PROJECTION.

Thoughts may be projected by following the last mentioned method (Distant Healing) and others will feel the effect of thought so sent forth, it being remembered always that no evil thought can ever injure another person whose thoughts are good. Good thoughts are always positive to bad ones, and bad ones always negative to good ones. One can, however, excite the interest and attention of another by sending him thought waves in this way, charging the prana with the message he wishes to convey. If you desire another's love and sympathy, and possess love and sympathy for him, you can send him thoughts of this kind with effect, providing your motives are pure. Never, however, attempt to influence another to his hurt, or from impure or selfish motives, as such thoughts only recoil upon the sender with redoubled force, and injure him, while the innocent party is not affected. Psychic force when legitimately used is all right, but beware of "black magic" or improper and unholy uses of it, as such attempts are like playing with a dynamo, and the person attempting such things will be surely punished by the result of the act itself. However, no person of impure motives ever acquires a great degree of psychic power, and a pure heart and mind is an invulnerable shield against improper psychic power. Keep yourself pure and nothing can hurt you.

(2) FORMING AN AURA.

If you are ever in the company of persons of a low order of mind, and you feel the depressing influence of their thought, breathe rhythmically a few times, thus generating an additional supply of prana, and then by means of the mental image method surround yourself with an egg-shaped thought aura, which will protect you from the gross thought and disturbing influences of others.

(3) RECHARGING YOURSELF.

If you feel that your vital energy is at a low ebb, and that you need to store up a new supply quickly, the best plan is to place the feet close together (side by side, of course) and to lock the fingers of both hands in any way that seems the most comfortable. This closes the circuit, as it were, and prevents any escape of prana through the extremities. Then breathe rhythmically a few times, and you will feel the effect of the recharging.

(4) RECHARGING OTHERS.

If some friend is deficient in vitality you may aid him by sitting in front of him, your toes touching his, and his hands in yours. Then both breathe rhythmically, you forming the mental image of sending prana into his system, and he holding the mental image of receiving the prana. Persons of weak vitality or passive will should be careful with whom they try this experiment, as the prana of a person of evil desires will be colored with the thoughts of that person, and may give him a temporary influence over the weaker person. The latter, however, may easily remove such influence by closing the circuit (as before mentioned) and breathing a few rhythmic breaths, closing with the Cleansing Breath.

(5) CHARGING WATER.

Water may be charged with prana, by breathing rhythmically, and holding the glass of water by the bottom, in the left hand, and then gathering the fingers of the right hand together and shaking them gently over the water, as if you were shaking drops of water off of your finger tips into the glass. The mental image of the prana being passed into the water must also be held. Water thus charged is found stimulating to weak or sick persons, particularly if a healing thought accompanies the mental image of the transfer of the prana. The caution given in the last exercise applies also to this one, although the danger exists only in a greatly lessened degree.

(6) ACQUIRING MENTAL QUALITIES.

Not only can the body be controlled by the mind under direction of the will, but the mind itself can be trained and cultivated by the exercise of the controlling will. That which the Western world knows as "Mental Science," etc., has proved to the West portions of that truth which the Yogi has known for ages. The mere calm demand of the Will will accomplish wonders in this direction, but if the mental exercise is accompanied by rhythmic breathing, the effect is greatly increased. Desirable qualities may be acquired by holding the proper mental image of what is desired during rhythmic breathing. Poise and Self Control, desirable qualities; increased power, etc., may be acquired in this way. Undesirable qualities may be eliminated by cultivating the opposite qualities. Any or all the "Mental Science" exercises, "treatments" and "affirmations" may be used with the Yogi Rhythmic Breath. The following is a good general exercise for the acquirement and development of desirable mental qualities:

Lie in a passive attitude, or sit erect. Picture to yourself the qualities you desire to cultivate, seeing yourself as possessed of the qualities, and demanding that your mind develop the quality. Breathe rhythmically, holding the mental picture firmly. Carry the mental picture with you as much as possible, and endeavor to live up to the ideal you have set up in your mind. You will find yourself gradually growing up to your ideal. The rhythm of the breathing assists the mind in forming new combinations, and the student who has followed the Western system will find the Yogi Rhythmic Breath a wonderful ally in his "Mental Science" works.

(7) ACQUIRING PHYSICAL QUALITIES.

Physical qualities may be acquired by the same methods as above mentioned in connection with mental qualities. We do not mean, of course, that short men can be made tall, or that amputated limbs may be replaced, or similar miracles. But the expression of the countenance may be changed; courage and general physical characteristics improved by the control of the Will, accompanied by rhythmic breathing. As a man thinks so does he look, act, walk, sit, etc. Improved thinking will mean improved looks and actions. To develop any part of the body, direct the attention to it, while breathing rhythmically, holding the mental picture that you are sending an increased amount of prana, or nerve force, to the part, and thus increasing its vitality and developing it. This plan applies equally well to any part of the body which you wish to develop. Many Western athletes use a modification of this plan in their exercises. The student who has followed our instructions so far will readily understand how to apply the Yogi principles in the above work. The general rule of exercise is the same as in the preceding exercise (acquiring Mental Qualities). We have touched upon the subject of the cure of physical ailments in preceding pages.

(8) CONTROLLING THE EMOTIONS.

The undesirable emotions, such as Fear, Worry, Anxiety, Hate, Anger, Jealousy, Envy, Melancholy, Excitement, Grief, etc., are amenable to the control of the Will, and the Will is enabled to operate more easily in such cases if rhythmic breathing is practiced while the student is "willing." The following exercise has been found most effective by the Yogi students, although the advanced Yogi has but little need of it, as he has long since gotten rid of these undesirable mental qualities by growing spiritually beyond them. The Yogi student, however, finds the exercise a great help to nim while he is growing.

Breathe rhythmically, concentrating the attention upon the Solar Plexus, and sending to it the mental command "Get Out." Send the mental command firmly, just as you begin to exhale, and form the mental picture of the undesirable emotions being carried away with the exhaled breath. Repeat seven times, and finish with the Cleansing Breath, and then see how good you feel. The mental command must be given "in earnest," as trifling will not do the work.

(9) TRANSMUTATION OF THE REPRODUCTIVE ENERGY.

The Yogis possess great knowledge regarding the use and abuse of the reproductive principle in both sexes. Some hints of this esoteric knowledge have filtered out and have been used by Western writers on the subject, and much good has been accomplished in this way. In this little book we cannot do more than touch upon the subject, and omitting all except a bare mention of theory, we will give a practical breathing exercise whereby the student will be enabled to transmute the reproductive energy into vitality for the entire system, instead of dissipating and wasting it in lustful indulgences in or out of the marriage relations. The reproductive energy is creative energy, and may be taken up by the system and transmuted into strength and vitality, thus serving the purpose of regeneration instead of generation. If the young men of the Western world understood these underlying principles they would be saved much misery and unhappiness in after years, and would be stronger mentally, morally and physically.

This transmutation of the reproductive energy gives great vitality to those practicing it. They will be filled with great vital force, which will radiate from them and will manifest in what has been called "personal magnetism." The energy thus transmuted may be turned into new channels and used to great advantage. Nature has condensed one of its most powerful manifestations of prana into reproductive energy, as its purpose is to create. The greatest amount of vital force is concentrated in the smallest area. The reproductive organism is the most powerful storage battery in animal life, and its force can be drawn upward and used, as well as expended in the ordinary functions of reproduction, or wasted in riotous lust. The majority of our students know something of the theories of regeneration, and we can do little more than to state the above facts, without attempting to prove them.

The Yogi exercise for transmuting reproductive energy is simple. It is coupled with rhythmic breathing, and can be easily performed. It may be practiced at any time, but is specially recommended when one feels the instinct most strongly, at which time the reproductive energy is manifesting and may be most easily transmuted for regenerative purposes. The exercise is as follows:

Keep the mind fixed on the idea of Energy, and away from ordinary sexual thoughts or imaginings. If these thoughts come into the mind do not be discouraged, but regard them as manifestations of a force which you intend using for the purposes of strengthening the body and mind. Lie passively or sit erect, and fix your mind on the idea of drawing the reproductive energy upward to the Solar Plexus, where it will be transmuted and stored away as a reserve force of vital energy. Then breathe rhythmically, forming the mental image of drawing up the reproductive energy with each inhalation. With each inhalation make a command of the Will that the energy be drawn upward from the reproductive organization to the Solar Plexus. If the rhythm is fairly established and the mental image is clear, you will be conscious of the upward passage of the energy, and will feel its stimulating effect. If you desire an increase in mental force, you may draw it up to the brain instead of to the Solar Plexus, by giving the mental command and holding the mental image of the transmission to the brain.

The man or woman doing mental creative work, or bodily creative work, will be able to use this creative energy in their work by following the above exercise, drawing up the energy with the inhalation and sending it forth with the exhalation. In this last form of exercise, only such portions as are needed in the work will pass into the work being done, the balance remaining stored up in the Solar Plexus.

You will understand, of course, that it is not the reproductive fluids which are drawn up and used, but the etheric pranic energy which animates the latter, the soul of the reproductive organism, as it were. It is usual to allow the head to bend forward easily and naturally during the transmuting exercise.

(10)   BRAIN STIMULATING.

The Yogis have found the following exercise most useful in stimulating the action of the brain for the purpose of
producing clear thinking and reasoning. It has a wonderful effect in clearing the brain and nervous system, and
those engaged in mental work will find it most useful to
them, both in the direction of enabling them to do better
work and also as a means of refreshing the mind and clearing it after arduous mental labor.

Sit in an erect posture, keeping the spinal column
straight, and the eyes well to the front, letting the hands
rest on the upper part of the legs. Breathe rhythmically,
but instead of breathing through both nostrils as in the
ordinary exercises, press the left nostril close with the
thumb, and inhale through the right nostril. Then remove
the thumb, and close the right nostril with the finger, and
then exhale through the left nostril. Then, without changing the fingers, inhale through the left nostril, and changing
fingers, exhale through the right. Then inhale through right
and exhale through left, and so on, alternating nostrils as
above mentioned, closing the unused nostril with the thumb
or forefinger. This is one of the oldest forms of Yogi breathing, and is quite important and valuable, and is well
worthy of acquirement. But it is quite amusing to the
Yogis to know that to the Western world this method is
often held out as being the "whole secret" of Yogi Breathing. To the minds of many Western readers, "Yogi
Breathing" suggests nothing more than a picture of a
Hindu, sitting erect, and alternating nostrils in the act of
breathing. "Only this and nothing more." We trust that
this little work will open the eyes of the Western world
to the great possibilities of Yogi Breathing, and the numerous methods whereby it may be employed.

(11)   THE GRAND YOGI PSYCHIC BREATH.

The Yogis have a favorite form of psychic breathing
which they practice occasionally, to which has been given
a Sanscrit term of which the above is a general equivalent.
We have given it last, as it requires practice on the part
of the student in the line of rhythmic breathing and mental

imagery, which he has now acquired by means of the preceding exercises. The general principles of the Grand Breath may be summed up in the old Hindu saying: "Blessed is the Yogi who can breathe through his bones." This exercise will fill the entire system with prana, and the student will emerge from it with every bone, muscle, nerve, cell, tissue, organ and part energized and attuned by the prana and the rhythm of the breath. It is a general housecleaning of the system, and he who practices it carefully will feel as if he had been given a new body, freshly created, from the crown of his head to the tips of his toes. We will let the exercise speak for itself.

(1) Lie in a relaxed position, at perfect ease.

(2) Breathe rhythmically until the rhythm is perfectly established.

(3) Then, inhaling and exhaling, form the mental image of the breath being drawn up through the bones of the legs, and then forced out through them; then through the bones of the arms; then through the top of the skull; then through the stomach; then through the reproductive region; then as if it were traveling upward and downward along the spinal column; and then as if the breath were being inhaled and exhaled through every pore of the skin, the whole body being filled with prana and life.

(4) Then (breathing rhythmically) send the current of prana to the Seven Vital Centers, in turn, as follows, using the mental picture as in previous exercises:

(a) To the forehead.

(b) To the back of the head.

(c) To the base of the brain.

(d) To the Solar Plexus.

(e) To the Sacral Region (lower part of the spine).

(f) To the region of the navel.

(g) To the reproductive region.

Finish by sweeping the current of prana, to and from head to feet several times.

(5) Finish with Cleansing Breath.

CHAPTER X.
SOUL DEVELOPMENT.

The Yogis not only bring about desired mental qualities and properties by will-power coupled with rhythmic breathing, but they also develop spiritual faculties, or rather aid in their unfoldment, in the same way. The Oriental philosophies teach that man has many faculties which are at present in a dormant state, but which will become unfolded as the race progresses. They also teach that man, by the proper effort of the will, aided by favorable conditions, may aid in the unfoldment of these spirit· ual faculties, and develop them much sooner than in the ordinary process of evolution. In other words, one may even now develop spiritual powers of consciousness which will not become the common property of the race until after long ages of gradual development under the law of evolution. In all of the exercises directed toward this end, rhythmic breathing plays an important part. There is of course no mystic property in the breath itself which produces such wonderful results, but the rhythm produced by the Yogi breath is such as to bring the whole system, including the brain, under perfect control, and in perfect harmony, and by this means, the most perfect condition is obtained for the unfoldment of these latent faculties.

In this work we cannot go deeply into the philosophy of the East regarding spiritual development, because this subject would require volumes to cover it, and then again the subject is too abstruse to interest the average reader. There are also other reasons, well known to occultists, why this knowledge should not be spread broadcast at this time. Rest assured, dear student, that when the time comes for you to take the next step, the way will be opened out before you. "When the chela (student) is ready, the guru (master) appears." In this chapter we will give you directions for the development of two phases of spiritual consciousness, i. e., (1) the consciousness of the identity of the Soul, and (2) the consciousness of the connection of the Soul

44

with the Universal Life. Both of the exercises given below are simple, and consist of mental images firmly held, accompanied with rhythmic breathing. The student must not expect too much at the start, but must make haste slowly, and be content to develop as does the flower, from seed to blossom.

SOUL CONSCIOUSNESS.

The real Self is not the body or even the mind of man. These things are but a part of his personality, the lesser self. The real Self is the Ego, whose manifestation is in individuality. The real Self is independent of the body, which it inhabits, and is even independent of the mechanism of the mind, which it uses as an instrument. The real Self is a drop from the Divine Ocean, and is eternal and indestructible. It cannot die or be annihilated, and no matter what becomes of the body, the real Self still exists. It is the Soul. Do not think of your Soul as a thing apart from you, for YOU are the Soul, and the body is the unreal and transitory part of you which is chang-.ng in material every day, and which you will some day discard. You may develop the faculties so that they will be conscious of the reality of the Soul, and its independence of the body. The Yogi plan for such development is by meditation upon the real Self or Soul, accompanied by rhythmic breathing. The following exercise is the simplest form.

EXERCISE.—Place your body in a relaxed, reclining position. Breathe rhythmically, and meditate upon the real Self, thinking of yourself as an entity independent of the body, although inhabiting it and being able to leave it at will. Think of yourself, not as the body, but as a spirit, and of your body as but a shell, useful and comfortable, but not a part of the real You. Think of yourself as an independent being, using the body only as a convenience. While meditating, ignore the body entirely, and you will find that you will often become almost entirely unconscious of it, and will seem to be out of the body to which you may return when you are through with the exercise.

This is the gist of the Yogi meditative breathing

methods, and if persisted in will give one a wonderful sense of the reality of the Soul, and will make him seem almost independent of the body. The sense of immortality will often come with this increased consciousness, and the person will begin to show signs of spiritual development which will be noticeable to himself and others. But he must not allow himself to live too much in the upper regions, or to despise his body, for he is here on this plane for a purpose, and he must not neglect his opportunity to gain the experiences necessary to round him out, nor must he fail to respect his body, which is the Temple of the Spirit.

THE UNIVERSAL CONSCIOUSNESS.

The Spirit in man, which is the highest manifestation of his Soul, is a drop in the ocean of Spirit, apparently separate and distinct, but yet really in touch with the ocean itself, and with every other drop in it. As man unfolds in spiritual consciousness he becomes more and more aware of his relation to the Universal Spirit, or Universal Mind as some term it. He feels at times as if he were almost at-one-ment with it, and then again he loses the sense of contact and relationship. The Yogis seek to attain this state of Universal Consciousness by meditation and rhythmic breathing, and many have thus attained the highest degree of spiritual attainment possible to man in this stage of his existence. The student of this work will not need the higher instruction regarding adeptship at this time, as he has much to do and accomplish before he reaches that stage, but it may be well to initiate him into the elementary stages of the Yogi exercises for developing Universal Consciousness, and if he is in earnest he will discover means and methods whereby he may progress. The way is always opened to him who is ready to tread the path. The following exercise will be found to do much toward developing the Universal Consciousness in those who faithfully practice it.

EXERCISE.—Place your body in a reclining, relaxed position. Breathe rhythmically, and meditate upon your relationship with the Universal Mind of which you are but an atom. Think of yourself as being in touch with All, and at-one-ment with All. See All as One, and your Soul as a part of that One. Feel that you are receiving the vibrations from the great Universal Mind, and are partaking of its power and strength and wisdom. The two following lines of meditation may be followed.

(a) With each inhalation, think of yourself as drawing in to yourself the strength and power of the Universal Mind. When exhaling think of yourself as passing out to others that same power, at the same time being filled with love for every living thing, and desiring that it be a partaker of the same blessings which you are now receiving. Let the Universal Power circulate through you.

(b) Place your mind in a reverential state, and meditate upon the grandeur of the Universal Mind, and open yourself to the inflow of the Divine Wisdom, which will fill you with illuminating wisdom, and then let the same flow out from you to your brothers and sisters whom you love and would help.

This exercise leaves with those who have practiced it a new-found sense of strength, power and wisdom, and a feeling of spiritual exaltation and bliss. It must be practiced only in a serious, reverential mood, and must not be approached triflingly or lightly.

GENERAL DIRECTIONS.

The exercises given in this chapter require the proper mental attitude and conditions, and the trifler and person of a non-serious nature, or one without a sense of spirituality and reverence, had better pass them by, as no results will be obtained by such persons, and besides it is a wilful trifling with things of a high order, which course never benefits those who pursue it. These exercises are for the few who can understand them, and the others will feel no attraction to try them.

During meditation let the mind dwell upon the ideas given in the exercise, until it becomes clear to the mind, and gradually manifests in real consciousness within you. The mind will gradually become passive and at rest, and the mental image will manifest clearly. Do not indulge in these exercises too often, and do not allow the blissful state produced to render you dissatisfied with the affairs of everyday life, as the latter are useful and necessary for you, and you must never shirk a lesson, however disagreeable to you it may be. Let the joy arising from the unfolding consciousness buoy you up and nerve you for the trials of life, and not make you dissatisfied and disgusted. All is good, and everything has its place. Many of the students who practice these exercises will in time wish to know more. Rest assured that when the time comes we will see that you do not seek in vain. Go on in courage and confidence, keeping your face toward the East, from whence comes the rising Sun.

Peace be unto you, and unto all men.

AUM.

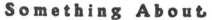

Something About
The Yogi Books

WHICH ARE A SERIES OF
UNIQUE WORKS ON
THE SUBJECT OF

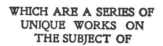

THE YOGI
PHILOSOPHY
══ AND ══
ORIENTAL
OCCULTISM

WRITTEN IN PLAIN
ENGLISH, AND SOLD AT
MODERATE PRICES

———

PUBLISHED AND SOLD BY

THE YOGI PUBLICATION SOCIETY
MASONIC TEMPLE. CHICAGO. ILL.

HATHA YOGA

THE YOGI PHILOSOPHY OF

PHYSICAL WELL-BEING

WITH NUMEROUS EXERCISES, ETC.

By YOGI RAMACHARAKA

Author of "Science of Breath," Yogi Philosophy and Oriental Occultism," Etc.

A Complete Manual of the Great Oriental Yogi System of Physical Well-Being—Health—Strength—and Vigor. It Preaches a Sane, Normal, Simple Theory of Physical Health, and tells how to put the theory into practice. It teaches that the Body is the Temple of the Soul, and should be kept clean and in good order. Its keynote is the healthy Man and Woman. Its purpose, the instruction and mankind to conform to the standard of that healthy man or woman.

Bound in Blue Silk Cloth, Lettered in Gold, 250 Pages.

Some time ago I bought a copy of your Hatha Yoga and I feel I must tell you how deeply I appreciate it, more than words can explain. It has been of great benefit to me. It is written so a child could understand and apply the teachings. Enclosed find money order for which I wish you would send me five more copies as I want to give them away. M. C. P. Spring Hull, Kans.

The Fourteen Lessons

THE HINDU-YOGI
Science of Breath

A Complete Manual of the Oriental Philosophy of Physical, Mental,
Psychic, and Spiritual Development by the Intelligent
Control of the Breath.

By YOGI RAMACHARAKA

I received the copy of "Science Breath" promptly and I am very
much pleased with it. The simple, clear, logical manner in which
it is written will certainly be appreciated and will enhance its use
fulness. Please send me another copy.—H. W. A., Pittsburg, Pa.

THE KYBALION

A STUDY OF

The Hermetic Philosophy of Ancient Egypt and Greece

BY THREE INITIATES

"The lips of Wisdom are closed, except to the ears of Understanding."

This new book is bound to attract the earnest attention of all students of the Secret Doctrines of the East. Perhaps the better way to describe this work is to give you the following words from its authors:

"From old Egypt have come the fundamental esoteric and occult teachings which have so strongly influenced the philosophies of all races, nations and peoples, for several thousand years. Egypt, the home of the Pyramids and the Sphinx, was the birthplace of the Hidden Wisdom and Mystic Teachings. From her Secret Doctrine all nations have borrowed. India, Persia, Chaldea, Medea, China, Japan, Assyria, ancient Greece and Rome, and other ancient countries partook liberally at the feast of knowledge which the Hierophants and Masters of the Land of Isis so freely provided for those who came prepared to partake of the great store of Mystic and Occult Lore which the master-minds of that ancient land had gathered together. In ancient Egypt dwelt the great adepts and Masters who have never been surpassed, and who seldom have been equaled, during the centuries that have taken their processional flight since the days of the Great Hermes. In Egypt was located the Great Lodge of Lodges of the Mystics. At the doors of her Temples entered the Neophytes who afterward, as Hierophants, Adepts, and Masters, traveled to the four corners of the earth, carrying with them the precious knowledge which they were ready, anxious, and willing to pass on to those who were ready to receive the same All students of the Occult recognize the debt that they owe to these venerable Masters of that ancient land.

THE KYBALION

The Hermetic Teachings are to be found in all lands, among all religions, but never identified with any particular country, nor with any particular religious sect. This because of the warning of the ancient teachers against allowing the Secret Doctrine to become crystallized into a creed. The wisdom of this caution is apparent to all students of history. The ancient occultism of India and Persia degenerated, and was largely lost, owing to the fact that the teachers became priests, and so mixed theology with the philosophy, the result being that much of the occultism of India and Persia has been lost amidst the mass of religious superstition, cults, creeds and "gods." So it was with Ancient Greece and Rome. So it was with the Hermetic Teachings of the Gnostics and Early Christians, which were lost at the time of Constantine, whose iron hand smothered philosophy with the blanket of theology.

THE HERMETIC PHILOSOPHY

"But there were always a few faithful souls who kept alive the Flame, tending it carefully, and not allowing its light to become extinguished. And thanks to these staunch hearts, and fearless minds, we have the truth still with us. But it is not found in books, to any great extent. It has been passed along from Master to Student; from Initiative to Heirophant; from lip to ear. When it was written down at all, its meaning was veiled in terms of alchemy and astrology, so that only those possessing the key could read it aright. This was made necessary in order to avoid the persecutions of the theologians of the Middle Ages, who fought the Secret Doctrine with fire and sword; stake, gibbet and cross. Even to this day there will be found but few reliable books on the Hermetic Philosophy. Although there are countless references to it in many books written on various phases of Occultism. And yet, the Hermetic Philosophy is the only Master Key which will open all the doors of the Occult Teachings!

ABOUT THE BOOK

"In this book we invite you to examine into the Hermetic Teachings as set forth in THE KYBALION. We therein give you many of the maxims and precepts of THE KYBALION, accompanied by explanations and illustrations which we deem likely to render the teachings more easily comprehended by the modern student, particularly as the original text is purposely veiled in obscure terms. We trust that the many students to whom we now offer this little work will derive as much benefit from the study of its pages as have the many who have gone on before, treading the same Path to Mastery throughout the centuries that have passed since the times of HERMES TRISMEGISTUS—the Master of Masters—the Great-Great. According to the Teachings, this book will attract the attention of such as are prepared to receive its Teaching. And, likewise, when the pupil is ready to receive the truth, then will this book come to him, or her, and not before. Such is The Law. The Hermetic Principle of Cause and Effect, in its aspect of The Law of Attraction, will bring lips and ear together—pupil and book in company. 'The Principles of Truth are Seven; he who knows these, understandingly, possesses the Magic Key before whose touch all the Doors of the Temple fly open.'—The Kybalion.

THE THREE INITIATES."

Bound in Blue Silk Cloth, Lettered in Gold, 223 Pages.

What is the Yogi Philosophy?

The Yogi Philosophy comprises the teaching which have come down the centuries of thought, investigation, experiment and demonstration on the part of the advanced minds of the Yogi Masters of India, Chaldea, Persia, Egypt and Ancient Greece—down to the present time—from Master to Student—Guru to Chela. It is the oldest philosophy in the world, although to the western world it comes as a new message—a Message from the East.

THE MASTERS

There have been in all ages certain highly developed, advanced and exalted souls in the flesh, known as the Yogi Masters and Adepts, although many of the tales told concerning them are myths, or pure fiction originating in the minds of some modern sensational writers. The Master Yogis have passed from lower to higher planes of consciousness, thus gaining wisdom, power and qualities that seem almost miraculous to the man of the ordinary consciousness. A Hindu writer speaking of them has said: "To him who hath traveled far along The Path, sorrow ceases to trouble; fetters cease to bind; obstacles cease to hinder. Such a one is free. For him there is no more trouble or sorrow. For him there are no more unconscious re-births. His old Karma is exhausted, and he creates no new Karma. His heart is freed from the desire for future life. No new longings arise within his soul. He is like a lamp which burneth from the oil of the Spirit, and not from the oil of the outer world." The Master Yogis are to pass through material obstacles, walls, ramparts, etc.; he is able to throw his phantasmal appearance into many places at once. He acquires the power of hearing the sounds of the unseen world as distinctly as those of the phenomenal world—more distinctly in point of fact. Also by his power he is able to read the most secret thoughts of others, and to tell their characters." Such are the Yogi Masters.

THE REAL AND THE IMITATION

The Western student is apt to be somewhat confused in his ideas regarding the Yogis and their philosophy and practice. Travelers to India have written great tales about the hordes of fakirs, mendicants and mountebanks who infest the great roads of India and the streets of its cities, and who impudently claim the title "Yogi." The Western student is scarcely to be blamed for thinking of the typical Yogi as an emaciated, fanatical, dirty, ignorant Hindu, who either sits in a fixed posture until his body becomes ossified, or else holds his arm up in the air until it becomes stiff and withered and forever after remains in that position, or perhaps clenches his fist and holds it tight until his fingernails grow through the palms of his hands. That these people exist is true, but their claim to the title "Yogi" seems as absurd to the true Yogi as does the claim to the title. "Doctor" on the part of the man who pares one's corns seem to the eminent surgeon, or as does the title of "Professor," as assumed by the street corner vendor of worm medicine, seem to the President of Harvard or Yale.

THE SCIENCE OF YOGA

There have been for ages past in India and other Oriental countries Yogi Masters who devoted their time and attention to the development of Man, physically, mentally and spiritually. The experience of generations of earnest seekers has been handed down for centuries from teacher to pupil, and gradually a definite Yoga science was built up. To these investigations and teachings was finally applied the term "Yogi," from the Sanscrit word "Yug," meaning "to join."

THE THREE FOLD PATH

Yoga is divided into several branches, ranging from that which teaches the control of the body, to that which teaches the highest spiritual development. Men are of varying temperaments, and the course that will best suit one will not be adapted to the requirements of another. One will seek progress and development in one direction, and another in a different way, and a third by a still different course. The Yogi Philosophy teaches that the way that seems to appeal the most to a man's general temperament and disposition is the one best adapted to his use at the present time. They divide the Path of Attainment into three paths leading up to the great main road. They call these three paths, (1) Raja Yoga; (2) Karma Yoga; (3) Gnani Yoga; each of these forms of Yoga being a path leading to the Great Road, and each being traveled by those who may prefer it—but all lead to the same place. We will now give a brief description of each of the three paths, which together are known to the Yogis as "The Threefold Path."

THE VARIOUS BRANCHES

Each branch of Yoga is but a path leading toward the one end—unfoldment, development, and growth. He who wishes first to develop, control and strengthen his physical body so as to render it a fit instrument of the Higher Self, follows the path of "Hatha Yoga." He who would develop his will-power and mental faculties, unfolding the inner senses, and latent powers, follows the path of "Raja Yoga." He who wishes to develop by "knowing"—by studying the fundamental principles, and the wonderful truths underlying Life, follows the path of "Gnani Yoga. And he who wishes to grow into a union with the One Life by the influence of Love, he follows the path of "Bhakti Yoga." But it must not be supposed that the student must ally himself to only a single one of these paths to power. In fact, very few do. The majority prefer to gain a rounded knowledge, and acquaint themselves with the principles of the several branches, learning something of each, giving preference of course to those branches that appeal to them more strongly, this attraction being the indication of need, or requirement, and, therefore, being the hand pointing out the path.

It is well for every one to know something of "Hatha Yoga," in order that the body may be purified strengthened and kept in health in order to become a more fitting instrument of the Higher Self. It is well that each one should know something of "Raja Yoga," that he may understand the training and control of the mind, and the use of the Will. It is well that everyone should learn the Wisdom of "Gnani Yoga," that he may realize the wonderful truths underlying life—the Science of Being—the scientific and intellectual knowing of the great questions regarding life and what lies back of life—the Riddle of the Universe. And it is well that everyone should know something of Bhakti Yoga, that he may understand the great teachings regarding the love underlying all life. The man best calculated to make general advancement along occult lines, is one who avoids running to extremes in any one of the branches of the subject, but who, while in the main following his own inclinations toward certain forms of "Yoga," still keeps up a general acquaintance with the several phases of the great philosophy. In the end, man must develop on all his many sides, and why not keep in touch with all sides while we journey along. By following this course we avoid one-sidedness; fanaticism; narrowness; short-sightedness and bigotry.

THOSE FOR WHOM THE TEACHINGS ARE INTENDED

Our books are intended only for those who feel an earnest attraction toward the higher teachings. They are for earnest students, inspired by the highest motives. Those for whom these teachings are intended will feel attracted to them. If you feel attracted toward these works, we will be glad to have you study them. If not we will feel just as kindly toward you, and will send you our best wishes for the hastening of the day when you will be ready for the advanced teachings. The matter is one entirely for the guidance of your Higher Self—let it decide for you. To those to whom a glimpse of the Inner Life has been given, the Yogi Philosophy will prove a treasury of the rarest jewels, and each time he studies it he will see new gems. To many it will be the first revelation of that which they have been all their lives blindly seeking. To many it will be the first bit of spiritual bread given to satisfy the hunger of the soul. To many it will be the first cup of water from the spring of life, given to quench the thirst which has consumed them. Those for whom this teaching is intended will recognize its message, and after it they will never be the same as before it came to them. As the poet has said: "Where I pass all my children know me," and so will the Children of the Light recognize the teaching as for them. As for the others, we can only say that they will in time be ready for this great message. Some will be able to understand much of the teaching from the first, while others will see but dimly even the first steps. The student, however, will find that when he has firmly planted his foot on one of these steps, he will find the one just ahead becoming dimly illuminated, so as to give him confidence to take the next step. Let none be discouraged; the fact that this teaching attracts you will in time unfold its meaning. Study it over and over often, and you will find veil after veil lifted, though veil upon veil still remains between you and That Beyond. Peace be to you.

ADVICE TO BEGINNERS

We advise interested beginners to study first our "Fourteen Lessons in Yogi Philosophy" which give a general outline of the entire subject. The beginner will also do well to study "Hatha Yogi" in order to render his physical body healthy and sound and thus give the Spirit a worthy Temple in which to manifest. "Science of Breath" may also be studied to advantage by the beginners.

As the student proceeds and develops in understanding he may take up the study of "Our Advanced Course;" then "Raja Yogi" and "Gnani Yoga" as his interest and desires dictate. Our little manual "Light on the Path" and "Illumined Way" will fit in well at this stage.

We will be glad to furnish inquirers with advice regarding the books they need, if they will ask us for the same. Each student of this subject, however, finds himself attracted to the books he needs—this is the Law. As the Teachers have written: "Know, O disciple! that those who have passed through the silence, and felt its peace, and retained its strength, they long that you shall pass through it also. Therefore, in the Hall of Learning, when he is capable of entering there the disciple will always find his master." And, so, the inclination toward the required book comes in due time.

FOURTEEN LESSONS

IN

YOGI PHILOSOPHY

AND

ORIENTAL OCCULTISM

By YOGI RAMACHARAKA.

Author of "Science of Breath," "Hatha Yoga," Etc.

An unique work covering the entire field of the Yogi Philosophy and Oriental Occultism, stating the most profound truths and hidden mysteries in the plainest, simplest, English style. No Sanscrit terms to puzzle the reader. Just the book you have been waiting for.

Bound in Silk Cloth, Lettered in Gold,———Pages.

A friend of mine loaned me a copy of your Fourteen Lessons and the teachings are just what I have been looking for since a child. They have brought me peace and happiness. I thank you sincerely for what it has done for me. M. E. A., Milwaukee, Wis.

The five books of Yogi Ramacharaka's that I have, I am very much interested in. Frederick J. M., Kingston, Ont., Can.

I have made a deep study of all your works and the good your books are doing is wonderful. With best wishes for your success, I remain Burd F. M., Omaha, Nebr.

ADVANCED COURSE

IN

YOGI PHILOSOPHY

AND

ORIENTAL OCCULTISM

BY YOGI RAMACHARAKA

Author of "Science of Breath," "Hatha Yoga," "Fourteen Lessons,"
Etc.

This books consists of Twelve Lessons, originally issued in monthly parts, treating upon the more advanced branches of the Yogi Philosophy and Oriental Occultism. It is practically a sequel to our book "Fourteen Lessons in Yogi Philosophy and Oriental Occultism," and continues the teachings of the "Fourteen Lessons," and leads the students to higher planes of thought, as well as showing him the deeper phases of occult truth. This book is intended only for those who feel an earnest attraction toward the higher teachings. It is only for earnest students, inspired by the highest motives. Those for whom these teachings are intended will feel attracted to them. If you feel attracted toward this work, we will be glad to have you study it, if not, we will feel just as kindly toward you, and will send you our best wishes for the hastening of the day when you will be ready for the advanced teachings. The matter is one entirely for the guidance of your Higher Self—let it decide for you.

Bound in Blue Silk Cloth, Lettered in Gold, 330 Pages.

To Yogi Ramacharaka.

Dear Teacher:—I must tell you that no other books or lessons have ever appealed to me like your own. A little more than a week ago the realization of my real self came to me and I am now a changed person. I have for some time had a certain intellectual grasp of the truth, but this is something so very different. It is wonderful and beautiful. Oh how grand it is to feel that you are master of yourself instead of slave of your passions.

H. R. E., Braddock, Pa.

HATHA YOGA

RAJA YOGA

The Yogi Philosophy of
Mental Development

By YOGI RAMACHARAKA

"Raja Yoga" is devoted to the development of the latent powers in Man—the gaining of the control of the mental faculties by the Will—the attainment of the mastery of the lower self—the development of the mind to the end that the soul may be aided in its unfoldment. Much that the Western World has been attracted to in late years under the name of "Mental Science" and similar terms, really comes under the head of "Raja Yoga." This form of Yoga recognizes the wonderful power of the trained mind and will, and the marvelous results that may be gained by the training of the same, and its application by concentration, and intelligent direction. It teaches that not only may the mind be directed outward, influencing outside objects and things, but that it may also be turned inward, and concentrated upon the particular subject before us, to the end that much hidden knowledge may be unfolded and uncovered. Many of the great inventors are really practicing "Raja Yoga" unconsciously, in this inward application of it, while many leaders in the world of affairs are making use of its outward, concentrated application in their management of affairs.

SYNOPSIS OF

The Advanced Course

LESSON I. Some Light on the Path. This lesson takes up an analysis of the little manual "Light on the Path," and explains in plain homely English the occult teachings so beautifully expressed in the poetical imagery of the Orient in the little manual.

LESSON II. More Light on the Path. This lesson continues the subject begun in Lesson I, and illuminates the secret wisdom so that the beginner is enabled to take the first steps on The Path intelligently.

LESSON III. Spiritual Consciousness. This lesson continues this wonderful explanation of "Light on the Path," and tells us of Spiritual Consciousness—"the flower that blooms in the silence that follows the storm"—Illumination.

LESSON IV. The Voice of the Silence. This lesson concludes the analysis and explanation of "Light on the Path," and tells us of the voice that proceeds from "out of the Silence that is Peace." A wonderful lesson.

LESSON V. Karma Yoga. This lesson teaches of that branch of the Yogi Philosophy that deals with the work of everyday life—the Yoga of Action. The true philosophy of work is given. This lesson is one much needed by the Western world.

LESSON VI. Gnani Yoga. This lesson takes up that branch of the Yogi Philosophy known as the Yoga of Wisdom. It gives the deeper teachings relating to the Riddle of the Universe, and the Absolute. Light on a perplexing subject.

LESSON VII. Bhakti Yoga. This lesson takes up that branch of the Yogi Philosophy known as the Yoga of the Love of the Infinite—of true religious feeling. It is as a cup of cold water to the thirsting soul. The true nature of Worship and Prayer is given.

LESSON VIII. Dharma. This lesson takes up the subject of Ethics and Right Conduct, as seen from the point of view of the Yogi Philosophy. It describes the origin of Ethics and Moral Codes.

LESSON IX. More About Dharma. This lesson continues the subject begun in the preceding lesson. It tells of the three-fold pillars of the Temple of Right Action—Revelation; Intuition or Conscience; and Utility or Human Law. The real meaning of Right and Wrong.

LESSON X. The Riddle of the Universe. This is a wonderful lesson. It gives the highest Gnani Yoga teachings. The Absolute and the Relative. The Infinite and the Finite. The Absolute and its Manifestations.

LESSON XI. Matter and Force. This lesson takes up the two great Manifestations, and shows the real nature of Matter and Force, and their relation to Mind, and to each other. A great scientific truth.

LESSON XII. Mind and Spirit. This lesson takes up the great Manifestation—Mind—and also the subject of the Atman or Spirit. The Universal Mind. Mind Substance. The relation between Mind and Spirit. The last of three wonderful lessons on the origin and nature of things.

A SERIES OF LESSONS

IN

GNANI YOGA

(THE YOGA OF WISDOM)

By YOGI RAMACHARAKA

This course gives the highest Yogi teachings regarding the Absolute and its Manifestations—the relations between the One and the Many—the Secret of the One Life—the Mystery of the Evolution of the Soul—the Law of Spiritual Cause and Effect—the Group-Soul—the Birth of the Ego—the Unfoldment of the Self—the Cycles of the Race—the Chain of Worlds—the Truth about Nirvana—the Divine Paradox—the Problem of Consciousness—the Reality and the Illusory—the offices of Will and Desire—the Future of the Race —the Past History of Man and the Races—the Adepts and Masters—the Brotherhoods—the Problems of Life—the Riddle of Existence. These and many other subjects of equal importance are taken up, explained and the dark corners illuminated. Some of the teachings to be given are entirely new to the general Western public, and partake of the nature of the Inner Teachings of the occultists.

Bound in Blue Silk Cloth, 302 Pages.

E. B., North Side, Pittsburg, Pa., writes she has just finished reading your book "Science of Breath," and considers it priceless.

I have studied many Occult and Mental Science works, but none of which ever developed Spiritual Illumination or produced that tranquil state of mind that I derived by studying the Yogi Philosophy.—N. R. B., New Zealand.

RAJA YOGA

Attainment of Power

But the follower of the "Raja Yoga" path is not content alone with the attainment of powers for either of above uses. He seeks still greater heights, and manages by the same, or similar processes, to turn the searchlight on concentrated mind into his own nature, thus bringing to light many hidden secrets of the soul. Much of the Yogi Philosophy has really been brought to light in this way. The practice of "Raja Yoga" is eminently practical, and is in the nature of the study and practice of chemistry—it proves itself as the student takes each step. It does not deal in vague theories, but teaches experiments and facts, from first to last. We give to our students, in our practical work on the subject of "Raja Yoga," (a work for which there is a great need in the Western world) full instructions "how" to do those things which have been stated to be possible by the numerous writers who had grasped the theory but had not acquainted themselves with the practice accompanying the theory.

Bound in Blue Silk Cloth, Lettered in Gold, 299 Pages.

THE INNER TEACHINGS OF

The Philosophies and Religions of India

By YOGI RAMACHARAKA

A COURSE OF TWELVE LESSONS

This is one of the most important of the several series of lessons by Yogi Ramacharaka, and will prove a worthy Final Message from this Great Teacher. It is wider and broader in scope and treatment than any of his previous works, as it covers the entire field of Hindu Philosophy instead of the conceptions and doctrine of but one of the many branches of the Oriental Teachings. To take up the many forms of the Hindu Philosophy and Religions, and to present them to the Western student in a plain, practical style, is quite an undertaking, but Yogi Ramacharaka pledged himself to make this work a success, and he always accomplishes that which he undertakes to do.

FUNDAMENTAL PRINCIPLES

In order thot you may understand the scope and field of these lessons, we herewith give you a brief synopsis of the subjects to be considered.

1. These lessons give you a plain, concise, but thorough synopsis of the Fundamental Principles of the Hindu Philosophies, which underlie the entire field of the Hindu thought, the understanding of which will enable any person of average intelligence to comprehend the various forms of the philosophical teachings of India, either in connection with the various religious denominations of that land, or else considered by themselves without reference to the religious creeds or divisions. Inasmuch as the Hindu Philosophies go to the very heart of human thought and speculation regarding the nature, origin, destiny and life of the universe, and what lies behind the universe, it follows that the principles of such philosophy must be

universal in their application and may be used in the consideration and examination of the philosophical or religious conception of any people, time, or land. A correct understanding of these principles will give you a "Touch-Stone" whereby the various speculations of the human mind, on those subjects, may be tested and tried, and their degree of soundness discovered.

THE INNER TEACHINGS

8. In addition to the full, clear and practical explanation and description of the various popular Philosophies and Religions of India, these lessons give a thorough consideration and description of The Inner Teachings of these philosophies and religions—the Esoteric or Hidden Side as well as the Exoteric or Outer Phase of the teachings which are given the general public. Under the surface of the Hindu Philosophies and Religions there is a great body of Inner Teaching which is rarely ever written or printed, but which is reserved for those sufficiently advanced to be able to comprehend it and among whom it is transmitted from mouth to ear. These lessons go into this hidden and secret phase of the teachings, by the means of which much light is thrown upon many obscure and perplexing points of the Outer Teachings.

DICTIONARY OF SANSCRIT TERMS

In the last lesson, the student is furnished with a Dictionary of the Sanscrit terms used in the lessons, which will aid him in the study of other works on the subject.

SPECIAL MONTHLY MESSAGE

Each lesson of this course contains a Special Message from Yogi Ramacharaka, addressed to his students, similar to those given in the lessons of several years ago, in the inspiring, helpful style so familiar to his earlier students. Each monthly Message, or Heart-to-Heart Talk, is accompanied by a Subject for Meditation and a Mantram of Affirmation, which the members of the earlier classes found so very helpful. This is the last course that will be probably issued from the pen of this Teacher, and these Messages will be in the nature of Farewell Advice and Admonition from him to his students.

Bound in Blue Silk Cloth, Lettered in Gold, 360 Pages.

I received the copy Philosophies and Religions of India and I understand that these are to be the last lessons. And indeed I feel that they are in truth last. The final analysis. I also feel and know that Yogi Ramacharaka's Eclectic System is the greatest that ever has or ever will be given to the world. The teachings from his pen I can only sum up in these words, supremely wonderful.
                            Yours fraternally,
                  Dr. Herbert Hoffman, Philadelphia, Pa.

THE SCIENCE OF

Psychic Healing

By YOGI RAMACHARAKA

A plain, practical series of lessons on Mental, Psychic and Spiritual
Healing, in its many phases and forms, with full instructions and directions regarding treatment, etc., very
little theory, but much practical instruction.

"All true healing results from an application of perfectly natural
laws and the power employed is as much a natural law as is electricity." Here is a partial list of subjects treated:

Natural Laws of the Body—How to Get Full Nourishment from
the Food You Eat—The Instinctive Mind—How the Body Carries
on Its Works of Regeneration—The Three Forms of Psychic Healing—The Principles of Pranic Healing—Yogi Teachers and Pranic
Healing 2,500 Years Ago—Laying On of Hands, Magnetic Heal-
ing, etc., During the Middle Ages—The Practice of Pranic Healing
—Means of Conveying Vital Force—Stroking, Rubbing, Kneading
and Massage—Breath Treatment—Pranic Breathing—Rhythmic
Breathing—General Directions—Pranic Treatments—How to Pre-
pare the Hands—Distant Healing—How Accomplished—Auto-
Pranic Treatments—Inhibiting Pain—Thought-Force Healing—
How to Apply It to Liver Troubles, Constipation, Rheumatism, the
Nerves, etc., etc.—Suggestive Healing—Practice of Suggestive
Healing—Self-Suggestion—Mental Healing—Metaphysical Healing
—Spiritual Healing—How to Become a Healer.

Pages.

Please extend to the writer of the Yogi Books my Soulfelt grat-
itude for the blessings received through his most beautiful teachings. They have prolonged my life on earth and given me a glor-
ious conception of "The absolute that fits me more perfectly for
life's unfoldments."—Mrs. B. G. O., Maple Rapids, Mich.

Mystic Christianity

OR

The Inner Teachings of the Master

By YOGI RAMACHARAKA

The mystic and esoteric Teachings are to be found burning as a bright flame in the heart of the Christian Religion. Many who have been reared in the Christian churches feel that surely the Truth must be found there, rather than in so-called "foreign religions," while many others have been erroneously led to believe that there was no Truth at all to be found in the Christian Teachings. For both of these classes this book is specially designed, although its interest will appeal to every student of philosophy, religion and occultism. The Truth IS to be found in the Christian Religion—all true occultists know this. Under the exoteric or commonly accepted forms of all religions there is always to be found an esoteric or hidden teaching—and Christianity is no exception to this rule. This is no new discovery—the early Fathers of the Christian Church knew this full well—the Gnostics taught Mystic Christianity—the Early Church was Mystic in its essence and inner circles. And all advanced students of Occultism, of whatever faith, venerate the Founder of Christianity, and find in His teachings a source of joy, delight and wisdom unknown to those who merely recognize the outer forms and teachings. This is why we feel so earnestly impressed to make public these Mystic Truths at this time. There is no reason for the Christian to forsake his faith and "run hither and thither after new gods"—he may find the very Truth imbedded in his own religion. Every true occult doctrine is contained there—every fundamental mystic truth may be found in Mystic Christianity if you but possess the key. There is but one TRUTH, and it is found in all religions, under the surface of the material doctrines. In the heart of the religion in which you were born and reared there is to be found the SACRED FLAME burning ever brightly, and subject ever to the Perpetual Adoration of the Spiritually Illumined. Those among you who have been prone to sneer at the teachings of Christianity shall see in these Inner Teachings the True Light of the Spirit—that those of you who have come to mock may remain to pray. Those among you who have sought an illumination outside of the Christian Teachings shall see the True Light burning on the Sacred Altar, and shall more than ever recognize the greatness, grandeur and godlike attributes of Him who has been known to the Wise of all lands and creeds as "The Light of the World." These things, and more, shall come to us who follow the Light of the Cross, as seen by those who know the Secret Doctrine—The Inner Wisdom— Mystic Christianity.

Bound in Extra Silk Cloth, Stamped in Gold—302 pages

Reincarnation

..and..

The Law of Karma

By

WILLIAM   WALKER   ATKINSON

A Study of the Old-New-World Doctrine of Rebirth and Spiritual Cause and Effect

This wonderful book embraces all the truths and knowledge of the foremost thinkers of the past and present on this interesting subject.

It was the universal belief a thousand years ago. Half of the world's inhabitants believe it to-day.

Every thinking person should read this great book.

Partial Enumeration of Contents:

What is Reincarnation?— The Egyptians, Chaldeans, Hindus, Greeks, Romans, Christians, Chinese, Japanese, Druids, etc., Idea of the Soul—Length between Incarnations— Where Does the Soul Dwell Between Incarnations?—What Happens at Death ?—The Great Astral World and Its Planes and Sub-Planes—Where the Soul Goes After Death and What It Does There—Rebirth and Its Laws—What Is the Final State of the Soul ?—The Message of the Illumined—The Justice of Reincarnation.—The Arguments for Reincarnation —The Proofs of Reincarnation—Arguments Against Reincarnation—The Law of Karma.

Cloth Bound; 256 Pages

Mental Influence

By

WILLIAM WALKER ATKINSON

—◆◆◆—

A Course of Lessons on Mental Vibration, Psychic
Influence, Personal Magnetism, Fascination,
Psychic Self-Protection, etc.

—◆◆◆—

—◆◆◆—

**Your money will be returned if any of these books
are not satisfactory**

Practical Psychomancy and Crystal Gazing

By

WILLIAM WALKER ATKINSON

———●●●———

A Series of Eleven Lessons on the Psychic, Phenomena
of Distant Sensing, Clairvoyance, Psychometry, Crystal Gazing, etc.

———●●●———

PARTIAL SYNOPSIS OF CONTENTS:

Scientific principles underlying Psychomancy. Sensing
objects by the Astral Senses. Projection of the Astral Body.

How to Develop Yourself. Development Methods. Concentration. Visualization. Psychometry. How to use the
Crystal and Mirror. General Instruction.

Simple and Space Psychomancy and their differences.
Seeing Through Solid Objects. Seeing Down Into the Earth.
Diagnosis of Disease by Psychomancy.

The Astral Tube.

Psychometry. Five Methods.

Various forms of Crystal Gazing. Directions of "How to
Do It," etc.

Astral Projection. What the Trained Experimentor may
do.

Space Psychomancy. What may be accomplished by
means of it.

Sensing the scenes, occurrences and objects of the Past, by
Astral Vision.

Future Time Psychomancy. Future events casts their
shadows before.

Dream Psychomancy. This lesson will explain many
instances in your own experience.

———●●●———

This most interesting study is stated clearly, so that all may
readily understand the fundamental principle of Psychic
Communication.

———●●●———